25 Aromatherapy Blends for De-Stressing

Excerpted from
The Aromatherapy Companion,
by Victoria Edwards

CONTENTS

Introduction:
Living with Stress

adapted from *Naturally Healthy Hair,*
by Mary Beth Janssen (Storey Books, 1999)

We now know that stress either causes or exacerbates a large percentage of all disease. Not only heart attacks, strokes, and immune system breakdowns but also almost every disease known has been linked to stressful toxins in our lives. How does this link work? Well, stress causes our body to release toxins. Toxins — those that our bodies produce when under duress as well as those that come from the food we eat and the environment that surrounds us — compromise our well-being. Work-family conflicts, financial pressures, and simply never having enough time are just a few of the many stressors we face every day.

The biological changes that take place in relation to perceived threats are called the stress response. Our bodies can adjust for and counteract the mild forms of stress that we encounter. In fact, stress can be good if we know how to use it to make things happen positively. Pressure can make us face up to challenges with extraordinary skill and fortitude. However, in the case of extreme, unusual, or long-lasting stress — emotional, physical, or chemical — our stress response and the ensuing control mechanisms can be quite overwhelming and harmful.

In prehistoric times, if a caveman out and about doing his hunting came upon a saber-toothed tiger, the alarm and fear that this created would begin the complex reaction called the fight-or-flight response, in which adrenaline and other stress-related hormones surge from the adrenal glands into the bloodstream. This response is designed to counteract perceived danger by setting in motion the body's resources for immediate physical activity. Our caveman's blood pressure would increase; his heart rate would rise; his immune system would be suppressed; his blood's clotting ability would increase; and his liver would dump stored glucose into his bloodstream, dramatically increasing blood sugar levels. He'd become superaware and feel quite strong. Our caveman would now be poised to put up a fight or run for his life. After surviving this ordeal, he'd need a period of time to recover before being faced with further danger. Having this "downtime" to recoup is the desirable way to handle stress.

Today, our bodies operate the same way. Times of stress produce the same biological and chemical responses, including the production of adrenaline. This adrenaline initially gives the body an energy boost. However, in large or frequent dosages, it can also make us feel anxious and nervous. It can create insomnia, depression, fatigue, headaches, digestive upsets, and downright irritability.

It is in facing unrelenting stress, as many of us do these days, that the possibility exists for the stress reaction to keep on humming along even after the fight-or-flight response has worn off. At this stage the adrenals secrete other hormones, such as cortisol and other corticosteroids, that, while necessary when the body is faced with emotional crises, can have very detrimental effects on our health if not controlled. They may increase the risk of a host of significant disease processes, including diabetes, high blood pressure, and cancer. These hormones also have immune system–depressing properties, which can set up conditions for a continuous string of maladies to take hold, from the common cold to allergies, gastrointestinal problems, and much more. In essence, if we can't manage the stress in our life, we are working our adrenal glands to exhaustion. In addition, this overload of hormones in the bloodstream overloads the kidneys and creates an internal buildup of toxins.

The Stress Epidemic

Stress can be defined as "the inability to cope with a threat, real or implied, to our well-being, which results in a series of responses and adaptations by our minds and bodies." Approximately 80 percent of visits to doctors are related to mind-body stress. The World Health Organization describes stress as a "worldwide epidemic."

—from the Wellness Councils of America

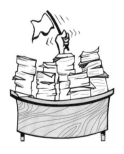

Using Aromatherapy

My first profound experience with aromatherapy occurred while treating a terrible sunburn — my own. I was in pain and had already tried various sunburn remedies, but nothing helped. When a blend of herbs and oils quickly brought soothing relief, it got my attention. I began to inquire into the properties of various oils and to explore their many possible applications.

Then at the age of 34 I contracted an infectious liver disease. It was a very frightening experience. I was severely ill, and my health remained fragile for many months after I had recovered from the most acute stage of the illness. It was during my recovery that I learned to trust in the profound healing power of essential oils. My liver had become so compromised during my illness that my body rejected food and medicines. I'm convinced that the essential oils I used during that time restored my liver to its full function.

There are so many different ways to use aromatherapy in your own life. Essential oils can be applied directly to the skin as part of a massage, reflexology, or meridian treatment. They can be dispersed in a bath, inhaled, or diffused into the atmosphere of a room. Specific oils affect specific systems throughout the body. You can target these various systems if you know how to select an essential oil for its properties, and how to select an effective and efficient means of delivery in each case.

EFFECTIVE APPLICATION TECHNIQUES FOR PARTICULAR BODY SYSTEMS

Essential Oil Application	Internal Organs and Systems Affected
Inhalation with diffusers	Respiratory, pulmonary
Internal uses; douches and boluses; suppositories	Digestive, eliminative, oral
Bath or spa therapy; massage and frictions; "aroma glows"	Works energetically on organ meridians
Algae, seaweed, and thalasso-therapy; herbal aromatic body wraps; poultices	Endocrine system
Inhalation with diffusers	Neurochemical responses
Subtle work; essences, crystals, color lights; homeopathy	Emotional responses

Airborne Scent

One of the miracles of aromatherapy is its absolute simplicity. Just a whiff of the right oil can adjust your attitude, clarify your thinking, steady your resolve, even ease your pain. I'm rarely without a small vial containing some blend to help me through the day. Lavender is often in my pocket for brief inhalations whenever stress is beating me down. A whiff of lemon invariably clears my head and refreshes my thought processes. Inhalations are a practical way to incorporate aromatherapy into your day.

JET LAG INHALATION

5   drops geranium essential oil
5   drops bay laurel essential oil
5   drops lavender essential oil

Combine the oils in a small glass vial with a tight stopper.

To use: Carry a vial in your pocket or purse while traveling. Sniff periodically throughout the day to forestall the exhaustion and brain fog of jet lag.

STRESS-BUSTER #1

Stress wreaks havoc on the immune system. This blend will help give it a healthy boost.

5   drops niaouli essential oil
5   drops ravensara essential oil

Combine the oils in a small glass vial with a tight stopper.

To use: Carry a vial in your pocket or purse and sniff periodically.

STRESS-BUSTER #2

This is a very calming blend.

5   drops lavender essential oil
2   drops Roman chamomile essential oil
34   drops ylang-ylang essential oil

Combine the oils in a small glass vial with a tight stopper.

To use: Carry a vial in your pocket or purse to sniff periodically throughout the day.

5   drops clove essential oil
3   drops nutmeg essential oil
10   drops sandalwood essential oil

Combine the oils in a small glass vial with a tight stopper.

To use: Carry a vial in your pocket or purse. If you're working at a computer terminal for extended periods, sniff periodically throughout the day.

The Aromatic Diffuser

There are many ways of scenting an environment. Incense has been used to deliver scent for thousands of years. More recently candle burners, simmering potpourri pots, and lightbulb rings have all become popular methods of dispersing scent atmospherically. Although these methods are aesthetically pleasing, they are not the best choices for aromatherapy. Commercial incense and potpourris are often rounded out with synthetic scents; their purity is unreliable. Additionally, incense smoke may transmit harsh, and even carcinogenic, chemicals along with its pleasing aroma. Candle burners and lightbulb rings can overheat delicate essential oils, changing their chemical makeup.

Diffusers act quite differently. Without altering or heating oils, they disperse them into the environment via an air-jet pump connected to a glass bell. A nebulizer within the glass bell diffuses a fine mist of negatively charged, scented ions into the atmosphere, much the same way that nature spreads fragrance.

The aromatic diffuser first appeared in Paris in 1960, when Dr. Bidault demonstrated the germicidal action of aromatic essences on tuberculosis, whooping cough, and influenza. His clinical observations indicated that disinfection of the air surrounding a patient had a therapeutic preventive effect. At the University of Paris School of Pharmacy, students tested his theories by collecting samples of air from an urban factory, the forest of Fontainebleau on the outskirts of the city, and a Parisian flat. By diffusing various essential oils into sealed chambers containing the air samples, they were able to validate the effectiveness of the essential oils against airborne bacteria and molds.

Diffuser Blends for De-Stressing

- **For colds and flu:** Oregano, lavender, eucalyptus, thyme, clove, cinnamon, peppermint
- **To calm:** Lavender, marjoram, geranium, chamomile
- **For nervous tension:** Lemon, orange, neroli
- **For meditation:** Clary sage, fir, cedar
- **For depression:** Bergamot, geranium, clary sage

The modern aromatic diffuser is a natural alternative to aerosol deodorizers and chemical air fresheners. A diffuser is a safe and convenient method of dispersing essential oils throughout a home, school, or workplace.

By using a diffuser, it is possible to dispense a therapeutic aromatherapy treatment to a number of people simultaneously. It is an excellent way of purifying the environment as well as administering the uplifting, rejuvenating, or relaxing effects of selected oils or blends to a group.

In the home environment, the therapeutic effects of diffused oils on the respiratory system are especially helpful during the cold and flu season, because the diffuser destroys airborne bacteria. When outside air is polluted, a diffuser can help create a safe, peaceful, and uplifting atmosphere indoors.

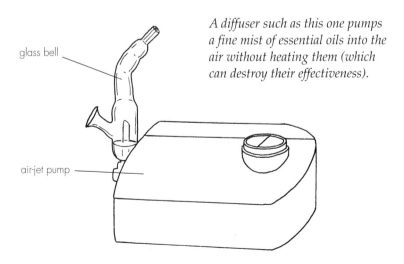

glass bell

air-jet pump

A diffuser such as this one pumps a fine mist of essential oils into the air without heating them (which can destroy their effectiveness).

ASTHMA WITH NERVOUSNESS AND ALLERGIES BLEND

- 5   ml (1 teaspoon) mandarin essential oil
- 5   ml (1 teaspoon) tarragon essential oil
- 5   ml (1 teaspoon) rosemary 'verbenon' essential oil

Combine the oils in a small, dark glass vial with a tight stopper and shake to mix.

To use: Use this blend in a diffuser during flare-ups of asthma. The blend can also be carried in a small glass vial in the pocket to be sniffed frequently throughout the day.

DETOXIFICATION BLEND

- 10   ml (2 teaspoons) lemon essential oil
- 5   ml (1 teaspoon) rose geranium essential oil
- 5   ml (1 teaspoon) everlasting essential oil

Combine the oils in a small dark glass vial and shake to mix.

To use: Use this blend in a diffuser when detoxifying or working on breaking a smoking, alcohol, or drug habit. This blend can also be carried in a small glass vial in the pocket to be sniffed frequently throughout the day.

RELAXATION BLEND

- 5   drops petitgrain essential oil
- 10   drops mandarin essential oil
- 20   drops lavender (*Lavandula angustifolia*) essential oil

Combine the oils in a small dark vial and shake to mix.

To use: Use in a diffuser to encourage relaxation.

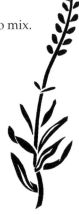

MEDITATION BLEND #1

- 4   drops myrrh essential oil
- 5   drops sandalwood essential oil
- 10   drops frankincense essential oil
- 2   drops clove essential oil
- 2   drops cistus essential oil
- 2   drops rose essential oil

Combine the oils in a small, dark glass bottle and shake well.

To use: Add to a diffuser and use to support meditation.

MEDITATION BLEND #2

- 10   drops clary sage essential oil
- 4   drops vetiver essential oil
- 2   drops cistus essential oil
- 20   drops cedarwood essential oil
- 5   drops fir essential oil

Combine the oils in a dark glass vial and shake well.

To use: Diffuse to support and enhance meditation.

Topical Applications

Most of us see the skin as a natural barrier. We imagine that not only does our skin hold us in, but it also keeps everything else out. We imagine that if our skin is unbroken, we present an impermeable surface, immune to the chemical stew of our environment. But the skin, our largest organ, is not impermeable. Acting more like a very fine sieve, our skin "breathes." As it inhales, it absorbs fine traces of the stuff on its surface; as it exhales, chemicals are excreted as fine components of sweat and sloughed-off skin cells.

The outer skin, made up of about 30 layers of cells, is called the epidermis. We shed dead skin cells every day. As the top layer of the skin dies off, a new layer is generated at the base. But as the skin ages, this process of cellular reproduction slows down. If the top layers are not sloughed off, the formation of new skin cells is slowed even further, and the complexion becomes tired and muddy-looking.

In 1968, researchers demonstrated the permeability of the human skin by attaching radioactive "tags" to chemicals in cosmetic preparations. The preparations were applied to the skin of human volunteers and the tagged chemicals were later identified in the volunteers' waste products. When I read, nearly 30 years ago, about this study, it changed my attitude about the ingredients I was putting on my skin.

I learned that essential oils placed on the skin are absorbed rapidly. In as little as 5 to 20 minutes an essential oil, applied topically, makes its way into the bloodstream, is carried to the lungs, and is exhaled with the breath. Essential oils are also eliminated through the skin, released in sweat through the pores, and released in urine through the bladder. As the essential oil travels through the body systems, tissues and organs benefit from its healing action.

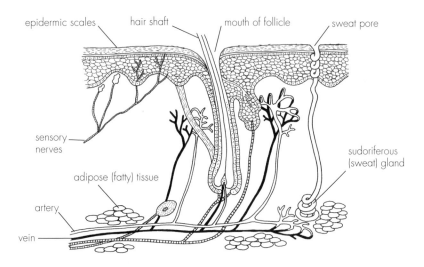

The skin both inhales and exhales particles. Essential oils applied to the surface eventually make their way into the muscles and bloodstream.

The Seven-Step Facial

Practiced weekly, this facial-care program will cleanse and revitalize a dull complexion, relax the mind, and nourish the soul. If you can open yourself to the present moment and the aromatic, soothing touch that these gifts from nature — herbs, flowers, essential oils, and other ingredients — can offer, then you can truly luxuriate in this spa experience.

1. Cleanse. Use the mild soap or cleanser of your choice.

2. Exfoliate. I keep a jar of homemade cleansing grains in my bathroom — a simple mixture of equal parts oatmeal, cornmeal, and ground almonds. Take about 1 tablespoon (15 ml) of the grains in the palm of your hand, add a little warm water to form a paste, and gently scrub your face and neck. Allow the grains to set on your face for a few minutes, then rinse with warm water, or rub off gently with your fingertips.

3. Steam. Heat a least 2 liters (2 quarts) of water to a simmer and pour into a large basin or bowl. Add 2 to 4 drops of an essential oil of your choice. Lean your face over the steaming water and drape a bath towel over the back of your head, forming a tent to capture the steam. Be careful not to burn yourself. Relax and let the fragrant steam engulf your head for 5 to 10 minutes.

A facial steam with essential oils added to hot water opens up the pores and soothes the soul.

Choosing Essential Oils for Your Skin Type

Skin Type	Recommended Essential Oils
Acne and congested	Thyme (sweet), neroli, bergamot, tea tree, spike lavender, sandalwood
Normal	Lemon, jasmine, rose, lavender, chamomile
Dehydrated	Carrot, rosemary 'verbenon', neroli, sandalwood, inula, everlasting
Oily	Melissa, lemon, lemongrass, basil, eucalyptus (E. radiata), camphor
Mature or wrinkled	Myrrh, frankincense, angelica, cistus, spikenard, violet, galbanum
Fragile, sensitive, or allergic	Bulgarian rose, blue artemis, blue chamomile, lavender

4. Massage. Gently *pat* your face dry — don't rub it. Choose a facial oil blend from the recipes listed in the following section and sprinkle a few drops into your palms. Rub your palms together and massage lightly over your face. Starting at the base of your neck, massage up the throat in a sweeping motion to your chin. From the corners of your nose, sweep under the cheekbones and up to your temples. Smoothing across your forehead, continue around your ears to the back of the neck, then down over your neck, shoulders, and bust area.

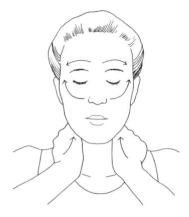

For the most effective massage, follow the paths indicated by arrows with the palms of your hands.

5. Mask. Choose one of the healing clay masks listed in the section beginning on page 14. Apply to your entire face and neck, avoiding your lips and around the eyes. Apply thickly to any areas congested with pimples or blackheads. Leave on for 20 minutes and then remove with a moistened washcloth.

6. Tone. Apply the toner of your choice (see pages 15–17) to clarify your complexion, close your pores, and remove any residual clay.

7. Moisturize. Top off your facial with a light application of a moisturizer or facial oil blend. In a few hours, your face will be glowing with health and vitality.

Facial Oils

Facial oils soothe and nourish the delicate skin of the face. They seal the skin, helping it retain precious moisture and providing protection from surface contaminants. They are also an important component of facial massage — by reducing friction, they prevent stretching and wrinkling of the skin. The delicate scent of the essential oils can also be quite relaxing and will linger with you through the day.

SENSITIVE OR INFLAMED SKIN LOTION

2	drops chamomile essential oil
2	drops neroli essential oil
7	drops sandalwood essential oil
5	drops bois de rose essential oil
30	ml (1 ounce) hazelnut oil

Combine all ingredients in a small, dark glass bottle and shake to mix.

To use: After cleansing and toning, place a few drops in the palms of your hands and massage lightly over your entire face.

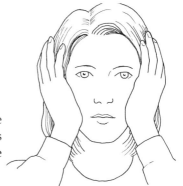

Apply facial oils gently, massaging with the palms of your hands.

AGING-SKIN LOTION

This wonderful facial formula supports cellular regeneration.

5	ml (1 teaspoon) sage essential oil
5	ml (1 teaspoon) rose geranium essential oil
5	ml (1 teaspoon) lavender essential oil
5	ml (1 teaspoon) rosemary 'borneol' essential oil

Combine all ingredients in a small, dark glass bottle; shake to mix.

To use: After cleansing and toning, place a few drops in the palms of your hands and massage lightly over your entire face.

OILY SKIN LOTION

10	drops niaouli essential oil
5	drops cypress essential oil
30	ml (1 ounce) hazelnut oil

Combine all ingredients in a small, dark glass bottle; shake to mix.

To use: After cleansing and toning, place a few drops in the palms of your hands and massage lightly over your entire face.

MOISTURIZING LOTION

3	drops vetiver essential oil
5	drops orange essential oil
10	drops lavender essential oil
30	ml (1 ounce) almond oil

Combine all ingredients in a small, dark glass bottle; shake to mix.

To use: After cleansing and toning, place a few drops in the palms of your hands and massage lightly over your entire face.

Clay Masks

Clay is one of the oldest of all skin treatments. Its cleansing and soothing properties were probably discovered by the women of ancient Egypt as they bathed along the banks of the Nile. Clay contains an abundance of silica and other mineral salts. Silica is a natural mineral that can take many forms and acts as a carrier of catalysts in chemical reactions. It is present in sand and glass and is found in the human body wherever hard edges appear, such as in the skin, nails, and hair.

Clay is a balancer and revitalizer. When applied to the skin as a mask, oxidation and circulation are accelerated, defensive functions are stimulated, and body temperature is raised.

Clay has certain little quirks that are important to know about. Dry clay powder can be stored easily. It is often sold in paper packaging, and no harm will come if dry clay is stored in plastic. However, as soon as water is introduced, the clay is activated; from this point it should come into contact only with organic materials. Ideally, this means mixing and storing in glass or ceramic vessels. Wet clay doesn't agree with plastic, and combining clays with metals can set off unpredictable and undesirable chemical changes.

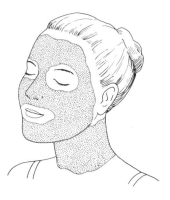

A healing clay mask draws out impurities and nourishes the skin.

Use wooden spoons or chopsticks for mixing and stirring, and make sure the water you are using is pure. You don't want to apply to your face a clay mask with bacteria growing in it! Distilled water is your best assurance of purity, but a reliable hydrosol (see page 18) or spring water can enhance the action of a clay mask. Measure your dry clay into a ceramic bowl and stir in enough water or hydrosol to form a soft paste. Add a few drops of an essential oil of your choice (3 to 5 drops per ounce of wet clay) and mix thoroughly. Apply to your entire face and neck, avoiding your lips and around the eyes. Leave the clay mask on until dry, then wash off with warm water or scrub off for an exfoliation treatment.

Use only healing clays found in health-food stores. The type of clay used for ceramics is not recommended.

- **Green clay** is an excellent all-purpose clay for healing and cleansing.
- **Rose clay** is highly absorbent and thus more drying. It makes a wonderful cleansing mask.
- **White clay** is very light and pure; used in its dry form, it is an excellent base for body powders.
- **Yellow clay** contains sulfur compounds. It is used to make clay packs to promote the healing of broken bones as well as to treat bone pain, sprains, and muscle aches and strains.

Astringents and Toners

Astringents and toners are an essential component of any successful facial-cleansing routine. They invigorate the complexion, remove any traces of soap, close up the pores, and quickly restore the skin's protective acid mantle (pH level). Here are several recipes.

BRISK TONER

10	drops lemon essential oil
7.5	ml (1½ teaspoons) apple cider vinegar
120	ml (4 ounces) distilled water

Combine all ingredients in a dark glass bottle. Shake well.

To use: Apply to the face and neck after cleansing.

CUCUMBER TONER

This is a wonderful formula for clarifying the complexion. Use it to feel crisp and clean during hot and muggy weather.

½	cucumber
15	ml (15 tablespoons) lavender hydrosol
30	ml (1 ounce) witch hazel
2	drops rosemary essential oil

1. Combine all ingredients in a blender and blend until the cucumber is liquified.

2. Strain through a coffee filter or cheesecloth. Put in a dark glass bottle with a lid and store in the refrigerator.

To use: Apply to the face and neck after cleansing.

Keep It Fresh

Any recipe that calls for fresh fruit or vegetable products will keep for only 2 or 3 days, even when refrigerated. Adding lemon juice or a few drops of rosemary essential oil will help preserve it. Make such recipes only in a quantity that you will use quickly, or share with your friends.

AROMA FRICTION

Using blends of essential oils with loofah scrubs or for brushing on dry skin is energizing and toning.

5	drops thyme essential oil
3	drops savory essential oil
12	drops MQV essential oil
90	ml (3 ounces) distilled or spring water

Combine the essential oils and water in a spray bottle; shake to mix.

To use: To stimulate and improve circulation, spray onto a loofah or body brush and scrub briskly over your body before or after a morning shower. Stimulate your meridians by working from the foot to the groin area, from the fingertips to the chest, and up the backs of your legs.

BODY TONIC

This is a wonderful tonic for skin that needs firming.

2	drops sage essential oil
12	drops lavender essential oil
10	drops rosemary essential oil
5	ml (1 teaspoon) glycerin or solubol
120	ml (4 ounces) rose water

1. Dissolve the essential oils in the glycerin or solubol.

2. Combine with the rose water in a spray bottle, and shake to mix.

To use: Use as a body spray, after bathing, or as an invigorating midday pick-me-up.

HERBAL TONER

235	ml (1 cup) distilled or spring water
30	ml (1 ounce) witch hazel
2	tablespoons each of the following herbs (dried): nettles, fennel, coltsfoot, marsh mallow, benzoin gum, comfrey, calendula, peppermint, orange blossoms, eucalyptus, chamomile, lavender, elderberries, lemon peel
12	drops lemon essential oil
12	drops lavender essential oil
30	ml (1 ounce) aloe vera gel
30	ml (1 ounce) glycerin

1. Combine the water and witch hazel in a small saucepan and heat to a simmer.

2. Remove from the heat, add the dried herbs, and allow the mixture to steep for 10 minutes.

3. Add the lemon and lavender essential oils to the herbal mixture and stir.

4. Strain the liquid through a cheesecloth to remove herbs. Add the aloe vera and glycerin.

5. Use a small funnel to pour the liquid into a dark glass bottle. Seal with a lid.

To use: Apply to the face with a cotton ball or pad to refresh the complexion and remove any residual soap or cleanser.

Hydrosols

Hydrosols (also called flower waters and hydrolats) are by-products of essential oil production, created during distillation. The waters used in the distillation process become naturally scented and impregnated with the plants' subtle water-soluble properties. Traditionally packaged in blue glass bottles in France, flower waters have been produced and used in cooking and cosmetics since ancient times in the Middle East, Tunisia, Egypt, and India. Jeanne Rose, executive director of the Aromatic Plant Project, has popularized herbal hydrosols in North America. She notes that this is a more accurate term than flower waters, as many are made from leaves, bark, or other parts of the plant.

The process of steam distillation using aromatic plants creates two complementary products: the essential oil and the hydrosol. Following the cooling of the aromatic gas, the oil-soluble components separate from the water. As they separate, they pass on part of their qualities and a small percentage of themselves: Maybe 2 to 10 percent of the essential oil ends up in the hydrosol.

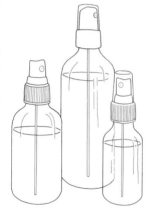

Hydrosols present themselves as perfect companions to such alternative health therapies as phytotherapy and homeopathy, and are excellent for people who are too sensitive to use essential oils.

Hydrosols are diffused with this type of pump bottle, often available in dark blue glass to protect the oils from sunlight.

CHOOSING THE RIGHT HYDROSOL

Skin Type/Use	Recommended Hydrosols
Normal skin	Neroli, rose, lavender, rosemary
Dry skin	Rosemary, orange blossom, rose
Oily skin	Melissa, lemon verbena, inula
Mature skin	Rose geranium, everlasting, rose
Eye compresse	Myrtle, elder flower, chamomile

Types of Hydrosols

Herbal hydrosols make excellent toners and skin refreshers. Those currently produced and commonly available in the United States and France include:

Bulgarian rose
Eucalyptus
Everlasting
Hyssop
Inula
Lavandin
Lavender
Lemon verbena
Linden
Melissa
Moroc rose
Myrtle

Neroli
Orange blossom
Peppermint
Rose geranium
Rosemary
Rosemary 'verbenon'
Thyme
Turkish rose

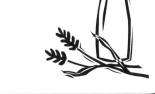

Applying Hydrosols

All hydrosols can be applied with a cotton ball or pad directly to the skin, or by misting 10 to 12 inches from the face with an atomizer. These bottles come in different sprays, from a fine mist to a squirt; choose one with a fine mist.

Hydrosols are perfect for use while traveling, especially during air travel, which is dehydrating. Hydrosols are also refreshing in the car and in drier climates, which dehydrate the skin. Occasional sprays have kept me awake during late, long-distance drives.

Hydrosols can also be used in making perfume, eau de cologne, and toilet water.

Hydrosol Blends

I created the following hydrosol blends while working in a skin clinic. They are the result of my own observation and study of the French concepts of skin care and hydrosol blending.

VELLEDA

- **30 ml (1 ounce) Roman chamomile hydrosol**
- **30 ml (1 ounce) rose geranium hydrosol**
- **60 ml (2 ounces) Bulgarian rose hydrosol**

Mix the waters together in a 120 ml (4-ounce) plastic spray bottle and shake.

To use: Misting the face with this blend works to rejuvenate on a deep cellular level. The effect is more profound with mature or aging skin. It is also good for very sensitive skin and imparts a natural glow.

HYDRA

- **30 ml (1 ounce) rosemary hydrosol**
- **60 ml (2 ounces) French lavender hydrosol**
- **30 ml (1 ounce) neroli hydrosol**

Mix the waters together in a 120 ml (4-ounce) plastic spray bottle and shake to make a rare and beautiful water solution.

To use: This blend is lovely for the skin and calming to the psyche; it maintains skin freshness if yours dries easily or if you live in a dry climate.

NAIAD

- **60 ml (2 ounces) lavender hydrosol**
- **30 ml (1 ounce) sweet thyme hydrosol**
- **15 ml (1 tablespoon) lemon verbena hydrosol**

Mix the waters together in a 120 ml (4-ounce) plastic spray bottle and shake.

To use: Naiad is useful for overactive sebaceous glands, blemishes, acne, and problem skin types.

DELPHI

- **30 ml (1 ounce) rose geranium hydrosol**
- **60 ml (2 ounces) lavender hydrosol**

Mix the waters together in a 120 ml (4-ounce) plastic spray bottle and shake.

To use: This blend is energizing, for a fast pick-me-up when you need to perform your best. It also rejuvenates the skin.

REJUVENATING BLEND

1   part rose geranium hydrosol
1   part rosemary hydrosol

This blend can be prepared in whatever quantity you need. Just mix together in a plastic spray bottle and shake.

SOOTHING BLEND

1   part lavender hydrosol
1   part thyme hydrosol

This blend can be prepared in whatever quantity you need. Just mix together in a plastic spray bottle and shake.

Water Therapy

Balneotherapy is the art of water therapy, and it is one of aromatherapy's best friends. There is nothing quite so soothing and relaxing as a leisurely soak in a hot bath. As the warmth of the water cradles your physical body, providing relief from the constant pull of gravity, your psyche is refreshed and restored, the weight of the world momentarily lifted. Add a few drops of well-selected essential oils and you approach nirvana.

Water is nature's greatest and most effective solvent. It acts as a liquid suspension, carrying a variety of minerals and chemicals, depending on its source. When we immerse our bodies in a warm bath, our skin rapidly begins to absorb chemicals that are suspended in the water. These chemical components can make their way to our bloodstream in as little as 2 to 15 minutes. It will take a normally healthy person from 30 minutes to 3 hours to eliminate most of these chemicals through the expired breath and urine. In unhealthy or obese people, this process may take up to 10 hours. That is why adding essential oils to a bath is such an effective aromatherapy treatment.

The premise of balneotherapy is built on this solvency. Just as we absorb the essential oils we intentionally add to the water, we absorb a variety of other chemicals and minerals suspended in the water. No two waters are exactly the same. Springwaters, often thought of as pure, actually contain a variety of minerals. It is the presence of these minerals, from the depths of the earth, that makes certain springwaters highly valued for their curative properties.

The amazing virtues of water have been sung throughout the ages. Ancient myths featured countless sea nymphs, mermaids, and water goddesses. It's no wonder that most ancient gods and goddesses associated with water were believed to be sources of life, fertility, and fecundity. Water is our element. We most likely evolved from aquatic creatures — and in any event, our first months of life are spent floating in an amniotic bath. In our dreams water symbolizes the ebb and flow of our emotions. We use water for cleansing, refreshing, and relaxing. Water is the basis for our body's evaporative cooling system. It flushes out toxic wastes, plumps up our cells, and lubricates our moving parts. Water is crucial to our survival. Without it we would literally dry up and blow away.

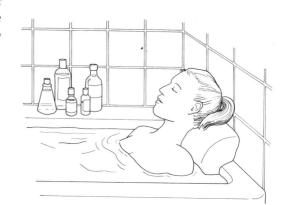

Bathing in waters scented with essential oils is one of the simplest and most enjoyable ways to enjoy aromatherapy.

A Brief History of the Bath

Although the Romans may not have invented the bath, they raised bathing to a high art. Roman citizens lingered for hours in communal hot baths, where they socialized, conducted courtship, and even sealed business deals. They built lavish baths wherever they found natural hot springs. The remains of Roman baths are still evident throughout Europe, the Mideast, and North Africa.

The Roman reverence for bathing has survived in Turkey, where patrons still visit public baths to be soaped, steamed, and scrubbed clean by attendants. Meanwhile, a highly ritualized bathing culture has evolved in Japan as well. Whole towns exist as destination resorts around Japanese natural hot springs. The harried Japanese make annual visits to these springs, and in between find time for frequent visits to the *sento* — the local communal hot-tub house.

With the fall of the Roman Empire, bathing fell out of favor in Europe. For the next few centuries the practice was considered suspect and unhealthy, immersion a frightening and distasteful experience. Washing was an unpleasant and infrequent necessity, to be carried out quickly and furtively, with a basin of cold water.

Water therapy as practiced today was introduced in Austria in the 19th century by the Reverend Father Sebastian Kneipp. Father Kneipp believed in the healing properties of water and prescribed treatments that included drinking mineral waters, soaking in hot springs, taking cold showers, and walking barefoot in the early-morning dew. Healing spas that subscribed to Father Kneipp's philosophy sprang up all over Europe, and "taking the waters" became a popular social pastime for the rich and privileged.

Today health spas abound throughout the Untied States, Europe, and the Mediterranean. Modern spas have evolved beyond mere mineral-water treatments to offer many other complementary therapies as well as physical fitness, relaxation training, and nutritional counseling. Aromatherapy has been universally adopted as a valuable synergistic component of most spa therapies.

Aromatherapy Baths

You can create your own spa experience with just a few oils and a tub of hot water. An aromatherapy bath is the ultimate luxury. Experiment with 3 to 5 drops of several different, complementary oils, adjusting the total amount to suit your individual taste. You can add the oils directly to the bath or, for added luxury, disperse them in a cup of milk first. On the following pages you'll find combinations of essential oils that you might try for the bath.

Other Bath Additives

Essential oils combine well with all other bath additives. Try adding any of the following to your aromatherapy bath:

- Epsom salts, sea salts, and algae to mineralize the water and increase buoyancy
- Oatmeal or honey to soothe and nourish the skin
- Bicarbonate of soda to "soften" the water
- Fresh or dried herbs and flower petals for their aesthetic and therapeutic qualities

---

☙ SOOTHE YOUR WORRIES AWAY ❧

Lavender essential oil
Chamomile essential oil
Geranium essential oil

☙ FLORAL ESCAPE ❧

Rose essential oil
Bois de rose essential oil
Ylang -ylang essential oil

☙ PAMPERED & SCENTED ❧

Bois de rose essential oil
Frankincense essential oil
Clary sage essential oil
Geranium essential oil

☙ LUXURIOUS SOAK ❧

Roman chamomile essential oil
Angelica essential oil
Neroli essential oil
Clary sage essential oil

☙ DEEP FOREST POOL ❧

Pine essential oil
Rosemary essential oil
Eucalyptus essential oil

☙ ESCAPE TO THE WOODS ❧

Sandalwood essential oil
Neroli essential oil
Cedarwood essential oil

☙ VITALITY ❧

Ravensara essential oil
Thyme essential oil
MQV essential oil

☙ VERY CALM NIGHT SOAK ❧

Marjoram essential oil
Cypress essential oil
Lavender essential oil

A Few Words on Water

Drinking and bathing in high-quality water is the most natural way to hydrate your body and preserve and promote your good health. Most tap water from public water supplies is loaded with chlorine, and often laced with other chemicals as well. Some of these chemicals are intentionally added to protect our health — fluoride, for example, is a highly controversial additive intended to harden children's teeth and prevent tooth decay — but other chemicals slip through in minute particles as traces of environmental pollution. If your skin is dry or irritated after bathing, and particularly if you notice a white residue on your skin, you might want to invest in a water filtration system.

Aromatherapy Massage

A well-selected essential oil formula enhances any type of massage or bodywork. There are many great books on massage, and hands-on courses are available in most major cities. I believe massage is best learned and practiced with another person. You can glean a lot of practical information from reading about it, but you need to feel and touch to really develop massage techniques. If you are inexperienced and feel insecure about giving or receiving a massage, I have included some tips to help you. Whatever the level of your massage training, aromatherapy can be added. By including essential oils, you will enhance the pleasure and therapeutic benefits of the treatment.

When using essential oils in a massage treatment, always choose oils that the person receiving the massage finds agreeable to smell. If you are going to experiment with your own blends, keep in mind that a 2 to 4 percent solution (7 to 20 drops of essential oil to each ounce, or 30 ml, of carrier oil) usually makes an appropriate concentration for a massage oil. Limit your blends to no more than three or four different essential oils. One ounce (30 ml) of massage oil is more than enough for an average massage, unless you are massaging a very large, dry, muscular, or hairy person.

Fatigue

Rosemary makes a great massage oil for fatigue, and it blends well with lavender and geranium. Rosemary oil must be diluted before applying to the skin. Add 20 drops to 1 ounce (30 ml) of carrier, or add 15 to 20 drops to bathwater.

ESSENTIAL OILS FOR DE-STRESSING

There are numerous ways to choose essential oils for massage. Because massage is such an effective way of transcending emotional barriers, I like to choose massage oils for their psychological effects.

Emotional Challenge	Essential Oils to Aid the Process
Anger (to soothe)	Chamomile, ylang-ylang
Anger (unexpressed)	Rosemary
Anxiety	Bergamot, citrus oils, melissa
Depression	Clary sage, bergamot, jasmine
Suicidal	Clary sage
Insomnia	Marjoram, neroli
Digestive trouble	Fennel, peppermint, cinnamon
Fear	Geranium, juniper, hyssop
Loss/death	Cypress, ud (agarwood), spikenard
Mental stress	Basil, citrus oils, neroli
Calming	Sandalwood, lemongrass, lavender
Physical pain	Ylang-ylang, clary sage, birch, pikenard
Oversensitivity	Mimosa, bois de rose
Spiritual, psychic protection	Frankincense, yarrow
Stress	Lavender, geranium, bergamot

Some Basic Massage Tips

- Make sure the room is a comfortable temperature. A warm, well-ventilated room is preferable. Music and soft lights or candlelight can enhance the atmosphere.
- Find a still point within yourself before you begin. Start by centering yourself, breathing evenly and deliberately. Feel your energy as it rises through your body, from your feet to your fingertips.
- Start slowly, using gentle, long, smooth, connecting strokes.
- Pay attention to muscle knots, constricted breathing, and soft sighs. Take note of painful spots as well as pleasure sites.
- Refrain from chatter. Follow your recipient's lead in conversation and don't be offended if she doesn't talk at all.

Aroma Points and Meridians

Electromagnetic nerve channels run all through the body. The energy of life, known in the East as *chi* or *qi*, runs along these channels, or meridians. Although chi is difficult to explain, it is real and can be felt. I have felt chi come through my hands while practicing Tai Chi. I have felt it shoot up my spine in deep yoga practice. The concept of this unseen and immeasurable energy, while new to the West, has ruled Eastern thought for centuries. Acupuncture treatments work on a knowledge of chi and its pathways.

The Chinese say that chi comes into the body with the breath, then flows through the twelve paired channels called meridians. These meridians can become blocked, and excessive heat or cold can deplete or cause excess energy. Through pulse diagnosis, these patterns can be understood. Symptoms are seen as specific expressions of an organ meridian's state of balance or imbalance. The acupuncturist's task, whether he uses needles or acupressure, is to rebalance the chi.

Volatile in nature and electromagnetic in composition, essential oils have important, subtle psychological and physiological properties. If you accept the concept of chi and acknowledge the healing power of essential oils, it becomes clear that essential oils influence the chi. Through study, conjecture, intuition, and practice, I have identified some specific oils for their balancing effect on the organ meridians.

I have also explored chi pulse correlations to specific patterns in music. For example, I have found that musical chords in the key of A major and in B major exert an influence on the gallbladder and liver meridians. The growing awareness and acceptance of vibrational medicine opens an exciting realm of possibility in the relationships of scent, sound, and color and their relationships to the meridians.

Essential oils are very powerful chemical messengers, that definitely affect the meridians. Even if you don't understand the concept of meridians or acupressure, you can benefit by rubbing your hands and feet with selected oils.

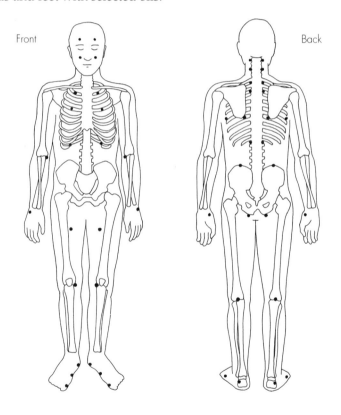

These diagrams show the location of meridian points (indicated by black dots) used in traditional Chinese medicine practices of acupressure and acupuncture to stimulate and balance the energy flow in corresponding areas of the body. Applying massage oils to these points can be beneficial as well.

There are numerous acupressure meridians on the face. The gall-bladder meridian starts at the outside corner of the eye, winds around the ear, and runs down the side of the head, tracing a shape like a Greek war helmet. Sinus and allergy problems originate here, and balancing this meridian can clear the sinuses and the eyes. The stomach meridian runs through the center of the cheek and nose area, all the way down to the feet. Dry lips and a stuffy, sometimes bloody nose are indications that the stomach meridian is out of balance. Some TMJ problems can be helped by balancing this meridian. The bladder meridian starts at the forehead, near the hairline over each eye, and runs straight back over the crown of the head to the nape of the neck. It continues down the back, where it splits into two forks that run all the way down each side of the spine. The small intestine meridian also runs through the face, along the smile line, from the corner of the nose down to the chin. Breakouts and rashes along this line can indicate food allergies and digestive or eliminative problems.

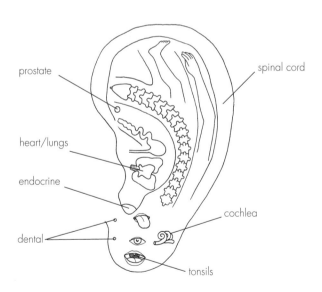

Meridians on the ear correspond to various organs and body parts.

Other meridians, such as the heart/kidney and spleen/liver, show up on the hands and feet instead of the face. However, all organs are represented on the tongue, in the iris of the eye, and in the ear points.

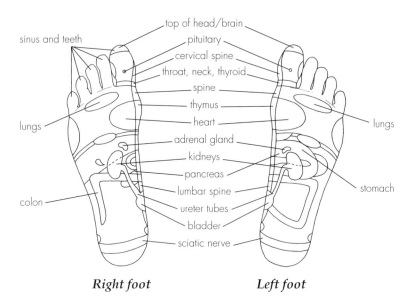

Right foot   **Left foot**

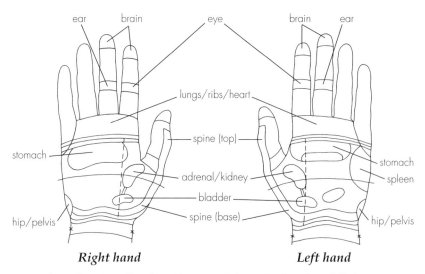

Right hand   **Left hand**

According to reflexology theory, points on the hands and feet stimulate corresponding body parts, as noted in these diagrams.

AROMATHERAPY FOR MAJOR ORGAN MERIDIANS AND CORRESPONDING EMOTIONS

Organ Meridian	Essential Oils*	Emotions/Attitudes
Lung/Large Intestine	Eucalyptus Inula Peppermint Pine	Grief and sadness. Possessiveness is the principal cause of grief and results in all kinds of accumulations such as cysts and tumors.
Heart/Small Intestine	Anise Lemon verbena Melissa Rose Ylang-ylang	Trying too hard, pretending you're okay when you're really not. You don't grow old from laughing! Joy is the positive side of all emotions.
Stomach/Spleen	Dill Fennel Kewda Roman chamomile	Fear. Where fear exists, love is absent. Where love exists, there is no fear.
Gallbladder/Liver	Lemon Neroli Peppermint Rosemary 'verbe-non'	Worry is payment on a debt never owed. Obsession, thinking too much, overanalyzing.
Kidney/Bladder	Cedarwood Geranium Juniper Sandalwood	Anger, resentment, bitter frustration. Encourages compassion and understanding. A deep laugh helps release anger and fears.
Umbilicus/Diaphragm	Frankincense Inula Lavender Spikenard Ud	A combination of all emotions. Fear of death.

*Use singly diluted or in combination of 2 or 3 oils.

Other Storey Books You May Enjoy

The Aromatherapy Companion by Victoria H. Edwards
The most comprehensive aromatherapy guide, filled with profiles
of essential oils and recipes for beauty, health, and well-being.

Hands-On Healing Remedies by Stephanie Tourles
150 recipes, using all-natural ingredients, to make your
own topical remedies to soothe everyday ailments.

The Herbal Home Spa by Greta Breedlove
A collection of easy-to-create personal care products that rival
potions found at exclusive spas and specialty shops.

Making Aromatherapy Creams & Lotions
by Donna Maria
101 recipes, using all-natural ingredients and following five
easy steps, to make your own creams, lotions, body rubs,
moisturizers, and lip balms.

Naturally Healthy Skin by Stephanie Tourles
A total reference for caring for all types of skin,
with recipes, techniques, and practical advice.

Organic Body Care Recipes by Stephanie Tourles
Homemade, herbal formulas for glowing skin, hair, and
nails, plus a vibrant self.

Perfumes, Splashes & Colognes by Nancy M. Booth
Step-by-step, illustrated instructions for making personal
blends with herbs, essential oils, and fragrance oils.

Join the conversation. Share your experience with this book, learn
more about Storey Publishing's authors, and read original essays
and book excerpts at storey.com.
Look for our books wherever quality books are sold
or by calling 800-441-5700.